How My Wife Saved Her Life

How My Wife Saved Her Life

By Lowering Her Diabetic A1C Level 8 Points In 8 Months

Paige E. Johnson, PhD

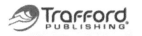

ISBN: 978-1-4269-5448-1 (sc)
ISBN: 978-1-4269-5449-8 (e)

Library of Congress Control Number: 2011900569

Trafford rev. 02/10/2011

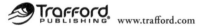 www.trafford.com

North America & international
toll-free: 1 888 232 4444 (USA & Canada)
phone: 250 383 6864 ♦ fax: 812 355 4082

Table of Contents

Introduction

This is the story of my wife, Sharon, who was gravely ill with undiagnosed diabetes; and her struggle to bring her diabetes in check and save her life. This book captures the process that my wife used (and still uses today) to lower her A1C level from 13.8 (14.0 the highest range) to 5.8 (normal range).

My wife was first diagnosed with Type II diabetes at age 51. Prior to age 50, she appeared healthy. She: began gaining weight from 140 pounds to 245 pounds; could not control her urination; had no energy; had extreme fluctuations in mood swings; had dry and flaky skin; was retaining fluid in her feet (including numbness and tingling sensations); had reduced mental cognizance; and was showing signs of being gravely ill. So, I took my wife to the doctor. The doctor diagnosed her symptoms were a result of a dangerously high A1C Diabetic Level (13.8), Fasting Blood Sugar Level (465), and that she had Type II Diabetes that demanded immediate treatment.

Here is a background synopsis leading up to her being diagnosed with Type II Diabetes. Previously, Sharon: did not get sick very often; would get a cold or sinusitis once a year; and bronchitis. Before she was diagnosed with Type II Diabetes, she developed: overactive bladder which is only a minor inconvenience; and elevated pressure in the eyes. The eye doctor began a glaucoma monitoring and prevention program due to the elevated eye pressure, a symptom of glaucoma and a complication often triggered by diabetes.

It was incredibly hot that year, particularly in August when it is supposed to be real hot. My wife, Sharon, could not tolerate the heat outside. Every time she started to go outside during the heat of the day, she got sick.

In August we had a lightning strike nearby our house. It blew out the television along with the satellite and did some other minor electrical damage. The repair people had to completely rewire everything. It took about six weeks to get everything working again. It was very expensive and very aggravating not having any television. It was very stressful between the extensive August heat and the lack on television. Nobody was happy being hot and without TV. My wife and I attributed her diabetic symptoms to be caused by stress, not diabetes.

At the end of August, I had to go out of town on business. Sharon went with me because I am in a wheelchair and if something were to go wrong, she would be there to assist. During the trip, it became noticeable that she was having medical problems with her overactive bladder condition. She was also incredibly thirsty. Although she saw one of her doctors before we left on the trip, she and the doctor attributed her symptoms to a stressful summer.

The trip was a real nightmare. Sharon would constantly be drinking water or going to the bathroom. She drank at least two 32 oz glasses of water in the morning, before or during breakfast. She drank one 32 oz glass of water between breakfast and lunch. She had a large diet soda plus another 32 oz glass of water for lunch. Between lunch and dinner, she polished off another 32 oz glass of water. When we went out to eat, the waiter had to bring us two pitchers of water plus the original glass of water for her to drink. After dinner and before bed, she would only drink half of the 32 oz glass of water so that she could sleep through the night without waking up too many times. That was a lot of water. Looking back, all that water probably saved her life.

When we returned, Sharon was feeling very ill. Sharon went in to see her doctor. She had lost 30 pounds while she was gone (three weeks). She and the doctor didn't know how. Sharon thought it was all the water that she was drinking. Her doctor tested her A1C

Diabetic Level and it was 13.8. The doctor told her that she had diabetes. The doctor immediately started her on a medical regimen in hopes to bring her diabetes under control. This included a gluconometer (blood glucose meter), medications, and diabetes education. Sharon cried most of that day about being diabetic.

Sharon visited the hospital diabetic education program nurse and the diabetic nutritionist. The hospital nurse took her blood sugar with the new gluconometer. Her blood sugar registered 465. It was still not even noontime. Sharon did not inform me that the nurse recommended that Sharon needed to go to the hospital emergency room. Sharon stated that she felt fine, did not need to be hospitalized, and refused hospitalization. Little did my wife realize how high her blood sugar had gotten and the related health risks. The nurse scheduled Sharon for diabetes education at the hospital.

Sharon went home to read about diabetes and how to lower her blood sugar. She looked forward to the diabetes education given through her local hospital. This began her journey towards lowering her systemic blood sugar.

Step One – Setting Priorities

Most people do not understand that diabetes will kill. It is not an acute disease, but a chronic disease. It does not send out high volume signals. It lets the high sugar in your body slowly and irreversibly, in some cases, poison your body. Diabetes is a vascular disease. It will become a tissue/organ disease. If left unchecked, it will destroy some part of your body in which the complications will kill you. Usually, though, diabetes will incapacitate your body in some manner. Blindness, heart disease, loss of a limb, or an increased chance of cancer will most likely occur before you die if you don't get your blood sugar under control. Not that any or all can still happen to you, but your odds of them not happening to you if you have good blood sugar will go DOWN, dramatically.

High blood sugar will kill you, but most importantly, it will slowly but surely restrict your lifestyle. We all know that the red blood cells carry oxygen and nutrients to the body. If our blood cells are sugar coated, we cannot get enough oxygen to various parts of the body. These parts cease functioning or deteriorate rapidly without oxygen and proper nutrients. The retina and optic nerve of the eye are particularly vulnerable. The heart needs oxygen to pump blood throughout the body. The brain, like all nerve tissue, is also extremely sensitive to oxygen deprivation. With diabetes, your organs are slowly suffocating. Some will go before others. Also, your ability to heal from cuts, abrasions, and infections is severely compromised. We all die. However, most people want to be able to enjoy a healthy life before we die.

Most of us want to be able to see, walk, and think. Don't think that you are without health concerns just because you currently do not have: major heart problems; vision concerns; current infections; or any other circulatory problems. With all the syrupy, sweet blood circulating in your body, depriving your body systems and organs of oxygen and vital nutrients; it is just a short number of ticks on the clock before major heath issues surface. Your body was in balance. Now, it is not. It is now time to evaluate your priorities and begin to get your body into balance. Life is a series of compromises. You have made too many detrimental compromises that result in hurting your body as you age. It is now time to make a choice to live. In order to live, you must take control of your health.

The A1C measures what percent of your blood is coated with sugar. The A1C number clearly states the percent of your red blood cells that are coated with sugar. For example, an A1C of 13.8 (like my wife) means that 13.8 percent of the blood is coated with sugar. Supposedly 15 percent and higher can be lethal to the body. Most healthy individuals, usually have an A1C of somewhere between 2 and 6 percent.

Sharon had just gotten through with seeing the eye doctor and telling him that she was diabetic and had elevated blood sugar. Her eye doctor was most concerned about this. He gave her prescribed eye drops to help protect her vision from degrading into full scale Glaucoma and possible blindness. Living had just seemed to be a chore to Sharon. She had not been happy about things, but now realized that her diabetes would likely destroy her vision if she let it. Sharon had to set priorities for her life. Seeing was one of the most important things to Sharon. Keeping her vision meant that she had to get her blood sugar under control – the sooner the better.

There is another myth that you can eat what you want and adjust your medication accordingly. Many of us believe that modern medicine has a pill for everything. We believe that the doctor just has to order a pill to make our physical problems go away. Many Type II diabetics believe that medication is the only thing they have to do to keep their blood sugar under control. **Medication is a necessity**. It is not the golden ticket to getting and keeping your blood sugar under control. One has to employ other strategies to getting the body healthy.

Medication, although a necessity, is hard on the liver and the kidneys of the body. The liver has to break down the medication so that the kidneys can filter it out. This is stressful on the body and can lead to liver function breakdown and kidney failure. However, without the medication, other systems can also fail, maybe even quicker. It is a balancing act that one must work out with one's own doctor.

My wife wanted to assist her body in lowering her blood sugar. During the course of the treatment and strategies that my wife has employed to assist her, she has cut the dosage of her medications by more than half and has deleted one medication in its entirety. Thus, this leaves her with two medications for her diabetes. These she will probably be on for the rest of her life. However, the stress on the liver and her kidneys has been significantly reduced.

You must decide whether or not to assist your body into getting healthy. Getting healthy and staying healthy is a lifetime effort, particularly for those who suffer from diabetes. When I talk about getting and staying healthy, I am not talking about not catching a cold or getting the flu. I am talking about keeping your body systems operating as best they can so that you keep your life, your vision, your limbs, and the ability to enjoy life for as long as you can.

Getting healthy will help fight off the colds and the flu that one occasionally gets. If you do get an illness, your body will be better able to fight off infections and the like. There is no guarantee that you will live for years. You could die in an accident, of have another non-diabetic health issue. However, this is about getting your body healthy and keeping it that way for a better quality of life. Your strategies should be something you can do now to become healthy. Then, you can decide what strategies to use to STAY as healthy as you can be.

We all have to set priorities. Everybody has to set their own. For physical priorities, usually, the number one priority for most is to live. The second priority is usually to live as healthy as possible. The third priority is to survive in this world economically. Then, family concerns can be met. Philosophical priorities such as God and country may come before or after any physical concerns. However, one cannot serve the philosophical priorities without being alive to do such. Even if you feel that family concerns are great and that job concerns are many, if you don't live and live healthy; you can't fulfill your other obligations to others. It is selfish of others not to let you take care of you. This even includes your family and your boss.

Sharon felt that if she had to live, her number one priority was that she had to see. Protecting her vision became my wife's overwhelming priority. That meant lowering her blood sugar and keeping it down.

Sharon read books and pamphlets on how to lower her blood sugar. She synergized the information that she read and tailored a strategy to meet her goals. There is no one strategy that offered her a solution. She combined strategies into six (6) steps. With the exception of Step One – Setting Priorities, the steps are not in order of importance. However, all the steps are important.

Just like a swimmer, you can swim only with your left arm or your right arm. However, if you use two arms, swimming is easier. Swimming is more efficient and more effective. If you choose to use your legs, swimming gets even more efficient and effective. So, take the plunge and use all the strategies that you can. Just like my wife, she used all the steps. If certain strategies compromise one or more of your major priorities – don't do it. If particular foods make you sick or can kill you, don't eat them. After all, it is YOUR life!

Step Two – Hydration Of Your Body

Other than taking a lot of medications, Sharon had to make some major lifestyle changes. One of the easiest strategies to begin for her was to drink lots and lots of water. The books and pamphlets tell you to drink 64 ounces of water a day. Healthy people are supposed to drink a minimum of 64 ounces of water, not fluid, not coffee, not soda, not juice, not milk, but WATER. Our bodies are supposed to be over 70 percent water. Drinking water helps to maintain the body fluids and cleanse the body of toxins. Her blood sugar was a toxin. She decided to routinely drink between 96 and 128 ounces of water every day. Yes, water.

Here in the United States we have an abundance of water throughout most of our states and territories. We have good, healthy drinkable water that flows out of almost every tap in nearly every American home. Drink it. Our Creator put it on this earth for nearly all animals and plants to consume. Water is the most basic part of all life on earth. Water is in nearly every food we eat and nearly everything we drink. It stands to reason that it should be one of the most elemental parts of getting one's body chemistry back into balance. Not only does water help the body and blood, but it usually helps the kidneys filter the wastes away from the body.

My wife and I hear the arguments. I don't like to drink water. I don't want to be going to the bathroom all the time. I'm too busy at work to drink water. I'm in school all day and can't get to the water. They are all excuses which might as well be that my cat has diarrhea and the house is upside down. If you want to heal your body and keep it healthy, drink water.

I don't know how many times a day that I see people walking around with some type of water bottle. Sometimes the water bottle is a commercial bottle that is packaged by a commercial company just like soda. It is almost a status symbol. Most of those bottles contain at least 16 ounces. Yet, people seem to go through at least 2 to 3 a day at work or at shopping without even thinking. My wife goes to the gym and nearly everybody has a 16 ounce water bottle that they drink and finish at the gym. That alone adds up to 3 to 4 16 ounce bottles of water, or nearly all what a healthy person should drink. If you add a glass of water or two for each meal, a glass of water with your medications, this put you at 80 to 106 ounces of water. Then, if you add a glass of water for 2 snack breaks and you are there (96 to 128 ounces) without working at it very hard.

Sharon fills a 32 ounce glass with water at least 3 times a day. She sips on it all throughout the day, including her meals and snacks. She takes a 32 ounce bottle of water to the gym and finishes it before she returns. Four times 32 equals 128 ounces, one gallon or two 2 litter containers of water. This does not include the added, under the tap occasional refill just because she is thirsty. What is your excuse?

Another excuse that people give about having to drink water is that they will only drink COLD ICE water if they have to drink water at all. Sharon has a hard time with ice cold water. She can't drink much at all. She can only drink a few sips and finds it uncomfortable to her stomach and body. It is mildly ok in the hot summer heat. But she can't physically drink the ice cold water very rapidly. Nor can she drink much of it, not even slowly. She finds that room temperature water is the easiest to drink. Not only that, it seems to satisfy her thirst better. I have seen her down nearly 16 ounces of water when she takes her medication.

Think about it. Your body is 98.6 degrees F. Ice cold water is 40 degrees or colder. Room temperature water is still cool at 70 degrees F. Your body does not have to heat it up but only a few degrees to get it into your body tissues. Your throat doesn't tighten up when you drink room temperature water and you don't get chills drinking room temperature water either. It works well for her. However, if you prefer cold water, get an insulated water bottle.

This strategy may not be just to your liking. Try it and see if you can get used to it. One more thought, water also helps to metabolize your food. It helps decrease your appetite. It takes the place of more expensive drinks. Last of all, it helps to rid the body of toxins, including, but not limited to sugar. Remember, what goes in must come out; and you must plan for your restroom breaks throughout the day.

I bet if the kidney failure patients could have consumed more water before they had kidney failure, they would have done so to prevent kidney failure from the body being dehydrated. I bet if people could remove or help decrease the effects of excess sodium on the body by drinking additional water, they would have done so before heart disease made its impact on the body. This is not to say that water will eliminate chronic systemic diseases, but I believe that eliminating/diluting the toxins within the body will allow the body to stay healthy for as long as it can.

Drinking water is painless and good for your body. My wife actually gets thirsty for water when she doesn't get her water in. You can't dislike water because it has little to no taste. What are you waiting for? Are you waiting to get sick or are you going to try to stay/get healthy? If you do sweat or you are extremely physically active, you might want to consider water that has electrolytes and is sugar free. You still need to drink just water. Not coffee, not beer, not tea, not soda, and not juice. Just like Samuel Cooleridge's *Rhyme of the Ancient Mariner*, "Water, water everywhere" but add "but plenty of drops to drink." Drink up, America! Drink up!

Step Three – Medications

Take your medications. They are there for a reason. They will save your life. For Sharon, the medications helped to reduce her blood sugar along with the other strategies. Your doctor will put you on prescribed medications. They are better than over the counter medications you can take. Over the counter medications may be helpful to borderline diabetics. You should tell your doctor about ALL the medications you are taking, including over the counter medications and vitamins.

Your vitamins and other over the counter medications may be taken at the wrong time and interfere with the absorption of your diabetic medications. Your doctor should know everything you are taking. Don't play Russian roulette with your health.

Sharon took her medications, to extend her life, and to save her sight. Getting her blood sugar down and getting it down quickly helped to save her sight. She realized that her high blood sugar had slightly damaged her eyes, her retina more specifically. She also had high cornea pressure. She had to get that pressure down so that her retina would sustain further damage to it. Retinas don't heal. Once damaged, they will always stay that way. Her priority was and still is to keep her sight for as long as possible. She knew that the only way to do this was to get her blood sugar down to normal levels – the quicker, the better. In addition, she had set aside the time to adhere to the eye doctor's strict eye health monitoring and Glaucoma preventive treatment program, that in all likelihood would not have been required if she did not have diabetes.

Part of taking your medicine is going to diabetes management training. My wife went and has gone to follow up training. During this training, multiple topics will be covered. Taking blood sugar readings was covered. A very brief discussion of blood sugar control medications, including insulin was also covered. This topic was not covered very well in my wife's class, at least not to her satisfaction. How to read and understand the nutrition labels on packages was also covered. A discussion on total carbohydrates per meal, per snack, and per day was covered. Taking care of your feet was also covered. However, in fairness to the diabetes management class, it was only two days. My wife feels that these topics and others really need at least five days of training. This is just as important as taking medications and doing all the other steps because this class will help you understand, at least the rudimentary beginnings, of how to deal with your diabetes.

Step Four – Exercise

Sharon decided that she needed to burn the carbohydrates in her body. Yet, she was overweight and could not handle hours of exercise. She did not have many exercise tools at home. Sharon did not feel that the house was conducive to motivate her to exercise. There were way too many distractions. Sharon belongs to a major gym in which she had purchased a lifetime membership years ago. This gym is not in our area. Sharon decided to join a gym that was close by. She looked into the costs and the programs that were offered and made a selection. The gym she chose has frequent group classes for cardio, weight lifting, and stress reducing programs. The gym she chose has both morning and evening classes. Yes, the gym has treadmills, free weights, and free standing exercise equipment in addition to the classes. She found a reasonably priced gym ($25/month) that was close to our house, offers a good selection of health programs (not just exercise), is clean, and offers a wide variety of different exercise classes – in addition to the treadmills, weights, and bikes.

Sharon goes to the gym nearly every single day. In the beginning, she would take one or two morning classes and then return at night for evening classes (totaling up to three hours per day). Because she was so overweight, she would also do the treadmill three times a week as a fat burner. She had to start slow because she was not used to walking quickly. She was also not used to walking far. In the weight lifting classes, she started with little to no weights. She has progressively worked up to nearly average weights. She doesn't do lunges nor do squats because of arthritic knees, but she will do leg strengthening exercises in their place.

Nearly everyone knows her or knows her face at the gym. She is a regular there. Sharon no longer goes for several hours a day. Instead she goes for one or two classes a day on most days (four to six days a week). During her first six months, Sharon did not lose a single pound. However, she did notice that her blood sugar was dropping dramatically. Within a month of exercising, her blood sugar had gone from the 465 to the mid-100s. This was good, but she was determined to do better.

Prior to this, Sharon would not leave the house except to run errands. She suffers from an anxiety disorder. One of the symptoms is that she doesn't like to leave the house. Yet, because she wants to see for as long as she can; she decided to get out and exercise. Exercise has benefits over and above that of lowering blood sugar. It also strengthens your heart, lowers your blood pressure, and helps lift your spirits. However, you have to exercise, not just think about it.

It is true that life is full of compromises. Job, family, PTA, Garden Club, hobbies, and whatever else fills your day. You have to make time for exercise. You must exercise nearly every day for at least one good solid hour. Everybody must be on board with this, including you. Sharon had a hard time finding the time. I, also, had to make a commitment to let her exercise when she took the time. It is better that she take the time to save her sight, and save her life.

Sharon didn't really have to give up much TV time. Our satellite receiver comes with a DVR or digital video recorder. This allows us to record the programs we really want to watch at OUR convenience. Our TV allows for rewind up to one hour.

Sharon did have to give up some of her reclusive nature to go exercise to save her eyesight. This was her major trade off. Exercise also gives her a snack, not a meal of snacks, but a snack. If she doesn't exercise, she may not eat her snack because she did not use the calories or feels that she deserves the extra carbohydrates. Sometimes, she has to snack, exercise or not, when she begins to feel dizzy or confused due to low blood sugar. Diabetics have to keep their carbohydrates in their bodies near low normal levels. This means that meals cannot be skipped and snacks must be anticipated and planned.

Family and children seem to be the biggest excuses people give for not exercising. If you were on chemotherapy or dialysis, your family would understand. Because you exhibit no major health symptoms, you and your family can make demands on your time. Remember, high blood sugar will lead to major systemic problems. You must keep it in check every day of your life. You must work at it every day.

Your children don't give up seeing their friends. You make them do their homework so that they will do well in school so that they can get a good job. Exercise is your homework. Your health is just as important. The children can do their homework on their own. They can learn to help out more around the house. You must learn to get well and stay well. This is no different than if they were sick, that you would make them take time out for their medicine. Exercise is your medicine as well. I notice a decline in Sharon's physical health (dizziness) and mental outlook on life when she misses exercise over several days.

Sharon exercises four to six times a week. There are weeks when she is sick or extra busy with errands when she exercises less. If she is too ill to exercise, she does not go. This is a rare occasion. In instances of great family distress or need, she also has to cut back on her exercise.

I realize that if she doesn't get to exercise on a regular basis, she may not be around long; and she may lose her sight. She helped me during my recovery. She got me out of the bed and into a wheelchair by herself until I could do it for myself. She did this and also took the time to go exercise. Yes, sometimes I had to wait. But now I am confident that Sharon will keep her sight and will be with me for years to come.

Life will always throw us curves. If my wife continues to exercise regularly, the few missed exercise days will have little effect on her overall well being. Her body won't notice the one to six days a month that she misses. I will have a wife that can see and won't need kidney dialysis for years to come, maybe hopefully never. There is no guarantee. At least she is doing all she can to see and get healthy, and I support her in her effort just as she supports me in mine to get healthy.

Step Five –
Diet Management

Weight control and food management are the next major concerns. Losing weight will help, but there are many thin and skinny diabetics in the world. Weight is not the most important issue. Losing weight should be a priority to someone who is overweight who is a food junkie like my wife is. Food is her drug. Just like alcohol is the drug of choice for alcoholics, food is the drug of choice for food junkies. Food is a legal substance for us. It is a necessary part of life. However, food junkies don't know when to quit eating nor want to. They want to eat just because it is there and it tastes good. Food junkies will not only eat to satisfy their tastes but will keep eating because it is comfort and feels so good to eat and eat and eat and eat. Food junkies also like large amounts of food. Food junkies will not only eat to satisfy a craving, but to eat multiple servings in one setting.

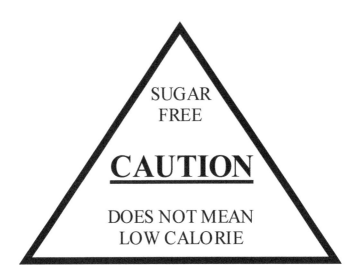

SUGAR
FREE

CAUTION

DOES NOT MEAN
LOW CALORIE

Food is basically comprised of protein (5 calories per gram), carbohydrates (5 calories per gram), and lipids (9 calories per gram) known to most of us as fats. We are not concerned with water in foods or minerals. Proteins help make up muscles and the enzymes that make up the inner workings of the body. Carbohydrates provide fuel for the body. Carbohydrates are not just sugars like sucrose, glucose and such. Starch is a carbohydrate. Alcohols are carbohydrates. Carbohydrates and fats may combine with protein to comprise body structures. Fats store energy and usually store the flavors found in food. Food is generally a composite of protein, carbohydrates, and fat. A balance must be struck between the three food components.

It would be nice if all food were just protein, just carbohydrate, and just fat. We could really watch our intake of the composition of the food we eat. Too much protein in the diet is hard on the kidneys. Too much fat consumed is hard on the circulatory system. Too much sugar is hard on the pancreas and hard on diabetics. My wife loved sugar – not only in donuts and candy, but in breads and pasta. She likes breaded fried chicken and rice. She likes vegetables, fruits, and juices. In short, my wife was not only a food junkie, but a true carboholic.

My wife had to get a living diet. Her diet must control the amount of carbohydrates she needs function but not contribute to her diabetes. A diet that controls the amount of protein she eats so that she does not destroy nor damage her kidneys. She must also control the amount of fat and lipids that she puts into her bloodstream so that her heart and circulatory system will stay healthy. My wife had to learn about foods.

A high protein and fat diet will give my wife lots to eat. The caloric intake can easily be watched and her carbohydrates will stay under control. The protein will break down into useable fuel for the body. The fat will also break down into useable fuel. However, this is not a healthy diet. Our Creator made our bodies to consume carbohydrates as well. My wife had to learn to pick and choose her carbohydrates and the type of carbohydrates that she feels is healthy for her condition.

A carbohydrate (carb) serving is 15 grams. We will call it a *carb serving* for short. According to the hospital dietitian, women get 3 *carb servings* per meal and men get 4. Mt wife continually complains that it is unfair for men to get 4 and women to only get 3. I tell her that life is not always fair. Diabetics get a morning and afternoon snack of one *carb serving*.

My wife read pamphlets of diabetic literature about foods. Most vegetable size servings are ½ cup to 1 cup per *carb serving*, depending on the vegetable. Some vegetables are *free carbs*. A *free carb* is that type of carbohydrate that one may consume without counting it in your carbarbohydrate intake. Most carbohydrates that are close to the ground and grown by the sun are *free carbs*. Carbohydrates such as celery, lettuce, broccoli, green peppers, radishes, beans, and such are generally *free carbs*. These she uses to fill up on. They are not exciting carbohydrates such as oranges, grapes, cherries, and watermelon; but they are filling and provide excellent sources of fiber. The fibrous carbohydrates are generally *free carbs*. Tomatoes are another source of *free carbs*. Tomatoes are low in calories and can be tasty in forms such as the whole tomato, spaghetti sauce, and salsa.

During her first three months, my wife decided to give up sugar, meaning sucrose. Nearly everything had to be sugar free. She uses sugar substitutes on cereal and in coffee. She and I were already diet soda drinkers. She gave up cakes and frosting and donuts. She did use bread and drank skim milk. She did not give up the sugar in these. Milk has sugar too. Lactose, the sugar found in milk and dairy products, contains one molecule of glucose and one molecule of galactose.

My wife read up on pasta and rice. She loves rice and pasta. However, what she read made her sad. Pasta and rice hit the bloodstream just like sucrose. Pasta and rice are jam packed of carbohydrates. It doesn't matter if the pasta is brown or multi-grained. It will hit the body just like sugar. However, don't despair there is a brand (Dreamsfield˚) of pasta that is only 5 grams of carbohydrates per serving as to 41 grams. It is not near as good as regular pasta, but it is pasta. Another alternative is spaghetti squash. My wife tried this. She is not a fan of this meal. There was not enough spaghetti sauce to cover the taste and texture of the spaghetti squash. Yet, some people like spaghetti squash. So this could be an alternative for them. My wife has yet to find carbohydrate friendly rice that she can eat. Therefore, rice is excluded from her diet.

Breads such as muffins, rolls, cereals, donuts, cakes and loaf breads are potentially harmful to diabetics. This is because they packed with carbohydrates. Not only is the wheat itself a carbohydrate; but, sugar is added to the mixture to make these wonderful delights. They are often packed with fat to give it moisture and wonderful flavor. Loaf white bread (sandwich bread) is high in carbohydrates (15 grams/slice) and high in calories (70-80 calories per slice). However, you can find good tasting loaf bread for 8 net grams of carbohydrates and 35 calories per slice. A *net carbohydrate* equals total carbohydrates listed on the nutritional label minus the grams of fiber listed on the nutritional label. Therefore, a food with 20 grams of carbohydrates and 5 grams of fiber equates to 15 grams of *net carbohydrates* or a one *carb serving*.

Nuts and berries are usually carbohydrate friendly. Do not eat nuts if you are allergic to this food. In fact, don't eat any food that which will give you an allergic reaction. Nuts release carbohydrates into the body very slowly. The body is usually able to handle these carbohydrates. Nuts can help lower blood sugar. The biggest problem with nuts is that a 1 ounce serving (just a small handful) is generally around 170 calories which does not help weight reduction. Nuts are also packed with fat. Berries are generally lower in carbohydrates than most fruit. One serving is usually a cup to a cup and a half. Wow! Berries taste good and can be rich in antioxidants. The problem with berries is that fresh berries are more expensive than fruits such as oranges and apples.

You can eat other fruits. Apples are high in fiber, but you must watch the size of the apple. Go ahead and eat the whole apple if you don't want to share the apple or can't share the apple. Apples don't stay good for long. They turn brown and get soft. Apples are a good source of fiber. Oranges must be shared or saved. You can only have a small part of the orange. If you like grapes, you get only 15 grapes per serving. That also means 15 raisins. It is important that you carefully watch the serving size. Don't just see a fruit and say that you can eat all you want. This is not true. Fruit juice is generally a no-no. Fruit juice is condensed fruit without the fiber or enough fiber to make a difference. Fruit is more satisfying to my wife than 2 to 4 ounces of fruit juice for a *carb serving*. However, if you want juice, have it. Just watch the serving size and nutritional information.

If you are a meat eater, your diet may include meat. This will help control your appetite because. Meat lasts longer in the digestive tract. This also helps fill the tummy. Meat will contain fat. Leaner cuts of meat should be used in diet. You can still have the higher fat meats like bacon, but treat it as a "special" dish and not for everyday or weekly use.

If you are not a meat eater, find ways to get protein, complete protein, in your diet. Whey protein is a way to enrich your diet. Whey protein added to water can be a good substitute. This will also contain carbohydrates. Well, you can't get around it. It will help with the hunger and help to balance out your nutritional needs. Our bodies need to obtain the essential amino acids that we cannot make for ourselves. These amino acids are found in proteins. The amino acids help make the enzymes and our body structures. Remember, life is a balance.

Fats and lipids (called fats) are generally overlooked. We need fats in our diet, but not a lot of them. First, fats help store the flavor that we enjoy in foods. Fats contain steroids and the hormones in foods. Some people refer to fat as that which is solid at room temperature and oils as that which is liquid. It doesn't matter; it is all fat. Fat is how the body stores energy for use later when we have used up our protein and carbohydrate stores. Oil helps to make our skin supple, our hair shiny, and combines with protein to make body structures. Fat intake should be kept to less than 30 grams per day, preferably less than 25 grams. Have fun!

My wife does have sucrose from time to time on purpose. She will have mini candy bars (5 grams of carbohydrates). She will occasionally celebrate a birthday or a wedding with a very small piece of cake with frosting. She treats sugar as a treat or special event. Two days a year she will splurge and not count sugar, calories, or carbohydrates. She does not drink alcohol much. She might have one to two drinks per year. Since she has been diabetic, I think that she has only had one glass of wine. Alcohol contains a whole lot of sugar. It is mostly sugar or carbohydrate. She feels that she would rather have the fruit instead of the fruity alcohol – each one to her own. Life is a compromise, find yours.

Learning to eat healthy is what it is all about. My wife tries to watch her caloric intake. She tries to make her calories healthy and not empty carbohydrate and fat calories. However, she still eats empty calories, but not like she used to. Empty calories will generally account for only 200 to 300 calories a day for her. Not perfect, but it is a start. She has lost and kept off nearly 50 pounds. She isn't losing anymore. Now she can walk without her back going into spasms. She has a bad knee due to arthritis aggravated by her past weight problem. Even her knees feel better with the weight loss.

My wife will always have a weight problem because she is a food junkie. She will always struggle with her weight. She has gone from a 3X size to a large. This is good. So far she has managed to maintain her weight. Exercise and caloric restriction help. She can only do so much. Her blood pressure is good usually 110 or lower over 70 or lower. Her cholesterol did initially rise to just over 200 after she got diagnosed with Type II diabetes. This happened because she ate lots of meat and eggs to help with hunger control without keeping a balance of foods in her diet. Now that she is on a cholesterol lowering drug and watches what she eats, her cholesterol has been 120 or lower. Her good cholesterol is in the "normal" range. The doctor has tested her liver and kidney functions. They have been well within the normal range. After three years, her A1C is 5.4. Below is a daily diet for my wife

BREAKFAST: a bowl of cereal (2 *carb servings*), 2-3 oz. skim milk (1/2 *carb serving*); one piece of toast with margarine and no sugar added jelly (1/2 *carb serving*), water (16 oz); and coffee with sugar substitute.

MORNING SNACK: apple (1 *carb serving*); 16 oz. water; and coffee with sugar substitute.

LUNCH: Sandwich with low carbohydrate bread with one slice cheese, one slice luncheon meat, and 2 teaspoons of low fat/low caloric spread or mustard (1 *carb serving*); one bag of chips 100 calorie dessert (1 *carb serving*); 16 oz of water; and a 12 oz diet soda.

AFTERNOON SNACK: Protein bar (1-1/2 *carb serving*) and 16 oz of water.

DINNER: 6 oz meat; a free carbohydrate vegetable; a serving of a starch vegetable (1 *carb serving*); 16 oz of water; a big bowl of berries and low calorie whipped topping (1-1/2 *carb serving*); and a 12 oz diet soda.

AFTER DINNER CRAVING: A bowl of sugar free jello with low calorie whipped topping (50 calories, no carbohydrates).

Step Six – Adequate Sleep

Diabetics, like everyone else, require adequate sleep. In my wife's case, this is 6-8 hours of sleep per night. Each person has their own requirement. Getting the required sleep helps my wife's diabetes. She does not get as dizzy (as she often does with lack of sleep); nor does she get as hungry when she has adequate sleep.

When my wife does not get adequate sleep, her morning normal blood sugar of 100-110 always fluctuates (higher or lower). If higher, her morning blood sugar is normally between 115 and 140. If lower, her morning blood sugar is normally between 60 and 80; thus, explaining her dizziness. In either case, lack of sleep affects her diabetes and increases her appetite for food.

Sleep helps to heal the body. Sleep reduces body stress. Sleep is a requirement for the body and a requirement which assists in keep my wife's morning, fasting blood sugar between 100 and 110.

Summary

Step One. Setting priorities is a must if you are going to take control of your life and control your diabetes. You must have a reason to control your diabetes. In my wife's case, her reason to control her diabetes is to save her eye sight and live a quality life in her old age. When it comes to prioritizing your time; hydrating your body, proper medical care, exercise, appropriate food choices, and adequate sleep must all be taken into account.

Step Two. Hydrating your body (64 oz to 128 oz per day) assists in controlling your diabetes.

Step Three. Obtaining medical care, health monitoring, diagnosis, and proper medications are essential in controlling your diabetes.

Step Four. Exercise not only assists in controlling your diabetes, but helps to make you healthier. Life is a balance. You must stay healthy and keep your body chemistry on an even keel if you want control your diabetes.

<u>Step Five</u>. Diet is probably the most essential factor affecting your diabetes. Sugar (carbohydrate) is the diabetic poison. Too much sugar in the body kills. It doesn't kill as fast as a bullet. It slowly debilitates the body, bit by bit.

<u>Step Six</u>. Adequate sleep assists in controlling your diabetes, stress, other illnesses, and general body health.

Conclusion

There are 25 million (and rising) diagnosed diabetics in the United States. Many are Type II diabetics. There are additional estimated 5 to 10 million undiagnosed Type II diabetics here in the U.S. That means that nearly one in ten people in the United States are diabetic and must manage their sugar and carbohydrate intake. It is estimated that one-third of the American population are obese. While not all obese individuals develop diabetes, obese individuals have a higher probability of becoming diabetics.

This should be a wake up call. Diet and exercise should be an important part of American life. We should encourage our schools and our businesses to encourage, if not mandate, physical activity time. Physical education and active recess should be a part of every school curriculum. Health insurances should help pay for gym memberships as a proactive health prevention program saving millions of dollars in future health care cost. People should be fighting over the rear parking spots in a parking lot as part of their exercise program, as to fighting for the parking spaces up front. If one needs to go up four or less stories in a building, one should take the steps if one is ambulatory rather than the elevator. People should do more walking. If people incorporate more physical activity in their normal daily functions, the time set aside for exercise should be reduced. However, life is a compromise.

Eating habits in all Americans should be changed. Vegetables, fruit, bread, cake, pasta, pizza, candy, and such are all fun to eat. Many carbohydrates are good for the body. The pancreas manages the blood sugar level. The pancreas will only last so long. Over a lifetime, the pancreas will handle only so much sugar in the blood.

Parents need to recognize that high sugar diets may not be good for them or their children. This includes fruit juices. Drink water, eat fruit, exercise, and get plenty of rest.

Life is a balance; and people should balance their life. My wife has had to make healthier comprises in an attempt to balance her life. Her blood chemistry has been altered significantly for the better because of her choices. We all talk about doing things healthier and better. It is about time that we do it.

Due to the changes in my wife's eating habits and lifestyle; I have done better in balancing my life. I watch my diet for calories as well as carbohydrates. I am obese and do not have: high blood sugar; high cholesterol; or high blood pressure. However, I am at higher risk to develop these health problems. I have lost weight myself (180 pounds). It isn't easy, but I do something.

American food manufacturers can do better at reducing the carbohydrate and caloric values of foods. Cake mixes can be lower in sugar. Cake frostings in a can should also be made in sugar free or no sugar added. Fiber, both soluble and insoluble fiber can be higher in foods. Breads can taste good and be lower in carbohydrates and sugar. However, let us not forget that foods such as cakes should be treated as "special" and not consumed every day.

Each one of us must learn to make healthier choices in both food and lifestyle changes. Otherwise, we will reach the day when 50 percent or more of the American population has diabetes. We will all be discussing the latest A1C values. We will all be taking some type of diabetic medicine. Many of us will go blind, be on kidney dialysis machines, have limb amputations, etc.

My wife has made considerable strides in managing her diabetes. She was diagnosed in her early 50s with diabetes. This is way too young for me to accept. We all need to be more aware of what we eat. We all need to take the time to exercise. We must become educated people when it comes to diabetes prevention. We need to take better care of ourselves. If we each take better care of ourselves, then maybe we can make Type II diabetes something that most of us gets when we turn 80 or 90, not 50 or younger.

My wife made poor choices earlier in her life. Now she makes better choices to ensure that she maintains her eye sight and has a better quality of life in her aging years. She has been and continues to be a success in managing her diabetes.

I am sharing the six step approach that wife used to save her life by successfully managing her diabetes. Her priority is that diabetes will not defeat her. Will it defeat you?

About the Author

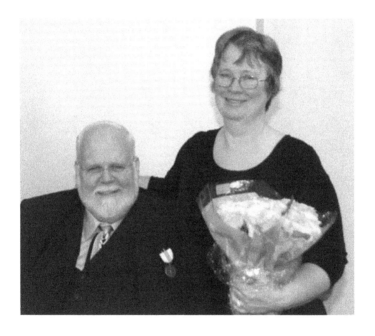

Dr. Johnson has a Doctorate and Bachelor's in engineering, a Master's in program management. Dr. Johnson is a highly recognized researcher, tester, evaluator, and developer with 40 years experience. He has documented his observations on how his wife saved her life after being diagnosed with diabetes.

Printed in the USA
CPSIA information can be obtained
at www.ICGtesting.com
LVHW041324210224
772445LV00005B/102